Congratulations,
YOU HAVE CANCER!

An empowering personal encounter
with breast cancer.

A positive, good feeling and spiritual approach on how to look at disease differently and recreate your experience of it!

Leslie Bishop

Outskirts Press, Inc.
Denver, Colorado

Congratulations, You Have Cancer!
An empowering, personal encounter with breast cancer.
A positive, good feeling and spiritual approach on how to look at disease differently and recreate your experience of it!

Outskirts Press
http://www.outskirtspress.com

ISBN-10: 1-59800-644-4
ISBN-13: 978-1-59800-644-5

Library of Congress Control Number: 2006931496

Outskirts Press and the "OP" logo are trademarks belonging to Outskirts Press, Inc.

Printed in the United States of America

An empowering, personal encounter with breast cancer, and a positive, good feeling, and spiritual approach on how you can look at disease differently and recreate your experience of it!

Appreciation and Gratitude

This book is dedicated to my family and friends who showed unconditional love and support through my whole experience with breast cancer.

I would especially like to thank my husband Bob, who I know has loved me long before we came forth onto this earth.

I would like to thank God/Universe for giving me the opportunity to experience breast cancer. The experience helped me to know and understand my own strength, power, and the ability I have within me to consciously create all my experiences!

I would like to thank Jerry and Ester Hicks/Abraham and Neale Donald Walsch, whose teachings and work have been such a huge inspiration in my life.

I would like to thank all my friends and family for offering their ideas for the front cover illustration— they were all great! A special thanks to Judy Bower, my friend since elementary school, whose idea was chosen to use for the front cover.

Appreciation and gratitude can be found within every moment, and when you become the observer of the moment, you will understand how miraculous every moment is!

—*Leslie Bishop*

Hope Is the Doorway

Hope is the doorway to belief, belief is the doorway to knowing, knowing is the doorway to creation, and creation is the doorway to experience.

Experience is the doorway to expression, expression is the doorway to becoming, becoming is the activity of all Life and the only function of God.

What you hope, you will eventually believe, what you believe, you will eventually know, what you know, you will eventually create, what you create, you will eventually experience, what you experience, you will eventually express, what you express, you will eventually become. This is the formula for all of life.

Home with God in a Life That Never Ends
Neale Donald Walsch

Preface

I have always known human beings are supposed to be happy and life was intended to be joyous and fun. Struggle and suffering are unnecessary and it is our choice how we choose to move through all experiences.

Do we see our glass as half empty or half full? When life throws us lemons, do we make lemonade? Do we see roses among the thorns?

Our perceptions form our reality.

"I see, said the blind man."

Disease

Disease knocks upon the door
Let it in
Embrace it
Do not be afraid
Welcome it
It is a teacher in disguise
Let it enlighten you
It fosters new understanding
Receive it
It is not the enemy
It is a friend
Let it share insights
Allow it
See the illusion you have created
Judge not
Let it be the arouser it was meant to be
Bless it
Send it on its way
It came to shake you and reawaken your soul!

—Leslie Bishop

Contents

Introduction

If you have been diagnosed or have been living with cancer of any kind, I would like to start off by saying, "Congratulations!"

How in the world could I say this to you or anyone else who has just been given such a diagnosis? The reason I say it is because I know the extraordinary message that is before you, just waiting to be received. This message is seeking your attention, and your encounter with cancer is one way to bring it to your awareness. I know what you are about to learn from your experience and from the sharing of my personal journey, and for this I am eager for you to read on.

I ask you to keep an open mind throughout this book. This openness could be the letting in of information that could change everything for you.

As you move through this text, my hope is that you will discover *why* you have gone through, or are going through, cancer. You will understand how it was created and how you can recreate your circumstances and be cancer free, if you so choose. You have an opportunity to look within yourself and ask some very important questions. It is in the *"asking"* that you will *"receive"* the answers.

I would also like to add, it is no coincidence you have chosen to read or look through this particular book. Because, you see, there is no such thing as a coincidence. Everything you experience in your life, even the choosing of a book, is governed by a Universal Law. This Universal Law is called "The Law of Attraction." It affects us on the physical and nonphysical plane, here on earth and throughout the Universe, and it is eternal. The Law of Attraction states: *"That which is like itself is drawn to itself."* So, your desire to want to know more has attracted you to this particular book at this particular time.

I would like to state upfront, I am not a medical doctor or health practitioner. I do not claim to be an expert in the field of cancer or any other diseases. The contents in this book are not medical recommendations for what you should or should not do. This dialogue is a recounting of my own experience and a recollection of what my intuition and knowledge have helped me to understand, over the years, about breast cancer. I am pleased and eager to be able to share it with you in this particular format.

The first few chapters briefly give an account of my own personal experience with breast cancer. The rest of the book focuses specifically on you and how you can recreate whatever it is you are going through.

Chapter 1
Signs!

It was time for my dreaded yearly gynecological exam. Getting it over with was the best part for me. It meant I had another whole year before I had to worry if any female problems were going on inside.

The doctor did his usual checkup and asked me if I had any discomfort or worries. I have always been healthy and right on track with my periods and did not have any concerns.

At the end of this particular visit, the doctor handed me a prescription to go and have a mammogram. Even though he did not feel any sort of lump in my breasts, he thought it would be wise to have one done. I had never had a mammogram before and thought it unnecessary since he checked me out and was not concerned. I stuffed the request for a mammogram in my wallet and went on my way.

Several months passed by. The news on breast cancer and how important it was for women to have a mammogram were in my face constantly after my visit. It seemed like everywhere I turned someone was being diagnosed with the disease. Still, I disregarded the request from my doctor and did not give it much more thought or attention.

One night, a couple friends of mine and I attended a fund-raising event in our community. There were several women speakers who got up and spoke to the group. One of the women stood up on a platform and spoke about her experience with breast cancer and how she had found a small lump in her breast while she was taking a shower. She begged the women in the audience to all have mammograms and emphasized how important early detection was in this matter. I thought it was odd that I kept hearing people talk about breast cancer and how I was seeing it all around me more so than ever. Still, I ignored the signs.

Another time, I was getting ready to pay for something at a store, and when I opened my wallet, a piece of paper I had folded up literally flew out of my purse and landed on the floor in front of me. When I reached down and opened it up, it was the request prescription the doctor had given me to go have a mammogram. This happened to me several times over the next few months. Still, I ignored the signs.

One night I was watching TV, and a special report came across the screen. Linda McCartney had died from breast cancer. For some strange reason the news report spoke loud and clear to my soul. The next day I made an appointment to have a mammogram.

"I have sent you nothing but angels."
—Conversations with God

Chapter 2
Victim of Circumstance!

"We have some news for you, Mrs. Bishop. Your mammogram is showing a mass about the size of a nickel. In fact, you can feel it right now. It is near the chest wall on your right breast," said the nurse who had just examined my x-rays.

"Are you serious?" I asked. What did I know? This was my very first mammogram.

"Well, let's take a look and see if we can feel it," she said.

She placed my hand on my chest wall by my right breast and damn, there it was, a nickel-sized lump.

"Oh, my God, this can't be real," I said, in disbelief.

I had never felt anything there before.

Well, okay, big deal, I told myself. *It's probably nothing anyway. I know I am healthy. I eat all the right foods and I exercise. I am in great shape. This can not be anything serious.*

My x-rays were sent to the doctor, where they were analyzed. A biopsy was taken from the existing lump, and it came back POSITIVE. It had been confirmed; it was cancer!

There was no big history of breast cancer in my family. How could this be happening?

When I heard the news I'd just been given, a fear like I have never felt seized my body and mind. Also, faith and hope emerged, as well. For a good part of my life, I'd been on the spiritual path. I had immersed myself in metaphysical classes and spiritual studies over the years, and I knew death was not something to fear. It is interesting how when you're faced with a grave situation, staying in your place of confidence and faith becomes a real challenge.

The doctor told me I had two options: they could do a mastectomy, which is to remove the entire right breast, or a lumpectomy, which is to just remove the lump. The doctor asked me which procedure I would prefer to have. For me, that seemed like an easy decision. I opted

Chapter 3
Angel in Disguise!

Chemo and radiation seemed to be the path to go down, but I wasn't so sure. I wanted to know what the right thing to do was. I needed to talk to someone, and I knew just who to turn to. I prayed, meditated, and talked to God. I talked to God a lot during this period of my life. I knew God spoke to us all the time through our thoughts and intuition, but it seemed as if the answer I wanted was not showing up. It seemed as if God was giving me the silent treatment. God was taking a vacation and it was on my time. What was the answer I wanted to hear? I wasn't even sure myself. All I knew was I did not want to go through chemotherapy.

Meditation seemed to work best for me. I would sit quietly every day for about fifteen minutes in silence. I asked God to help me come up with an answer. What I kept receiving in my thoughts was that *"It really didn't matter what I decided to do, chemo or no chemo, either choice would be okay."* At the time, I did not understand exactly what that meant. My inner knowing, my intuition, was saying one thing, and the doctors were telling me another. After a while, you begin doubting your intuition and go with what everyone else around you is telling you to do.

A decision was made, and I opted to do both chemotherapy and radiation at the same time. I wanted to get the whole ordeal over and knock it all out as quickly as possible. The doctor scheduled my treatments to begin in a couple of weeks.

Those two weeks felt like years. I was nervous and scared; eventually it manifested itself one Sunday afternoon following a church service. The service had come to an end, and I fought to hold back my tears. It seemed like a losing battle; I broke down and started to cry. A few friends gathered around, wanting to know what was wrong. I explained to them how nervous I was about going through the chemotherapy treatments and how horrible I felt about it all. This was poison I was going to be injected with. I wanted them to understand this poison would be destroying and killing everything inside me that it touched and it may even kill me as well. I explained to them how I couldn't imagine this toxic substance going through me, when all of my life I had taken good care of myself and now I was subjecting my body to this merciless toxin.

Within moments, I felt a comforting arm reach across my shoulder. It was a friend who stayed after church and who had taught me in a class, on several occasions, about how powerful our thoughts and beliefs are and how they can affect our circumstances and create our reality.

She said to me, in a comforting tone of voice, *"Leslie, why don't you just change your thought about all of this?"*

Confused and perplexed, I asked, *"What do you mean?"*

She said, *"Instead of thinking of the chemo as killing everything in your body that it touches what if you thought about it as **renewing and healing** everything it touches?"*

Wow, I had never thought about it in that way.

She reminded me how powerful our thoughts are, and how all of our thoughts are conscious energy. She continued on, saying that with each thought we think, over time, we will attract what we are thinking into our experience. She reminded me what we had learned over the years together in our classes, but I had completely forgotten. I was too afraid and caught up in my own fear.

WOOO WHOO, you would have thought someone just handed me a million dollars. I struck it big, and it was just the number I needed. I had won the lottery in that moment!

Of course, I knew better. I know how powerful our thoughts are. I know how every thought we think produces a feeling inside us, and the feelings send out energy, and by the law of attraction we will create exactly what we believe to be true. If I thought and felt the chemo was going to harm me, then my body would respond to that thought and I would attract it as my experience. If I believed it would renew and heal me, then I could have that experience instead.

God sent me the answer I had been praying for and it was through a friend, an earth angel, a message of hope and a light at the end of the tunnel. Not only did we end up laughing about the whole thing, we decided to call it "clean-o-therapy" instead of "chemotherapy." She also had me call her whenever I needed her for support through my whole ordeal. Her name was Pamela, and I will be forever grateful.

This is how **awesome** God/Universe is. Every person who comes into our life is an angel in disguise. We have to start recognizing them and listen to the messages they have for us. Messages are always coming our way; do we just "listen" or do we really "hear"?

There are many messengers on our path, and we are never walking alone. Become aware of who is playing a role in your life, and listen carefully to the words they are speaking. Everyone is mirroring to you what you are asking for, whether it is positive or negative; they are showing you to yourself. They are there to help you recreate your circumstance. They may just be the answer to your prayer!

"Keep away from people who try to belittle your ambitions. Small people always do that, but the really great make you feel that you, too, can become great."
—Mark Twain

Chapter 4
My Circumstance, My Creation!

Sitting in the chemo chair was challenging for me. Every couple weeks I would go for treatments. The room seemed morbid and chilly. Glancing around at the other people who were in the same room was similar to walking into a funeral parlor. The energy was not exciting nor was it any fun. Everyone looked so hopeless and scared. Their facial expressions were depressing, as if they were saying, *"Look what life has done to me. I am a victim of this circumstance, and there is nothing I can do about it."* I could relate to them because I had almost gone to the same place in my thoughts as well. I hoped by just being in the same space that my optimistic energy would send out comfort and peace to them so they, too, could move to this place of empowering thought.

I started to feel better about my situation. I realized I needed to embrace my circumstance, but not at the cost of giving up hope. I didn't feel I had to, as a lot of people say, *"fight"* the disease. Why would I fight something I believed had no power over me? I know when you push against or resist something, you only make it part of your experience. When you embrace a situation and you love it, you can love it to death. It actually loses its power over you. So I stayed focused on the moment at hand and made the best of each chemo and radiation session I went to.

There is nothing better than a good song or good music to uplift your spirits. Music has always helped me to relax and feel joyful and free. It seems to transport me and take me away from fearful thoughts and worries about life. So I carried with me to all of my chemo sessions a CD player and played uplifting music. This was a tremendous tool for allowing my well-being to flow. I knew how important creative visualization was, and so, as the music was playing, I would visualize the chemo as a blue-green liquid running through my veins.

The color blue-green is a very healing color. I would see it renewing my body and everything it touched. It was cleansing, healing, and rejuvenating me. The old cancer cells were dissolving, and new healthy cells were being born again.

I visualized the roots in my scalp and my hair as being strong and healthy. My hair was going to hang in there with me for the ride. I figured a few of the strands would stray, but the majority would have to stay put. I knew God would be pushing me too far if I were to lose all my hair. That's where I drew the line. (Lots of ego, I know.)

I started to challenge myself with the whole process. I knew I could do it. I knew who I was and that I was more powerful than my circumstance. I did not talk much about what I was going through to other people. I knew the more I talked about it, if it didn't feel good, then I was just going to be adding to the negative energy and giving it more power. I was a co-pilot with God, and we were going to reroute this flight and travel in a new direction!

I felt good most of the time, and I did not lose my hair. It thinned a bit, but no one would have ever known I was going through chemo and radiation all at the same time. I knocked out the chemo and the radiation treatments within six months. I did get nauseous a couple of times after some of the treatments, but I asked doctors for some medication to help ease the queasiness, and it did help.

There was a short time in the middle of the treatments when I wanted to stop. I felt like the first few were enough to cleanse and heal me, but after discussing it, my husband Bob coached me to keep going. It was the more promising path to take.

I reevaluated my thoughts and started to look at the whole thing as a race to the finish. If I quit now, I would be letting myself down. Proudly, I crossed the finish line and felt like a champion for staying in the game. This was even before Lance Armstrong!

My doctor was amazed at how well I was doing and how I looked through the entire process. I felt good and had an abundance of energy. I took up Bikram yoga, which helped energize my body, flush out toxins, and rejuvenate my cells. I believed yoga freed up the blocked energy within me, therefore improving my energy flow.

After the whole ordeal was finished, I decided to attend a breast cancer support group. It was nice to be with other people who had gone through similar experiences. I wanted to share my story and hear what other women had experienced. What I found out about this group was interesting. We all told our story and relived the whole experience. Some women in the group had gone through breast cancer decades ago and were still talking about it. They talked mostly about the fear around it and how they *still* feared it may return. I honestly was thrilled to be done with the whole ordeal; I could not imagine it coming back into my experience again. I realized this was a subject I did not want to keep talking about. I was ready to move on and thought this group would be able to help me to do that. But, this particular group was stuck; most were still stuck in the fear of it all. I wanted to feel good about the whole experience and my future, so I made a decision to move forward and depart from the group, and I did!

I had a lot of time to wonder about my life. I started to look within myself. It was interesting for me to think about why experiences were showing up for me in this particular way. Why had this all been happening to me? I became more in touch with my intuition and the small, still voice within. I found myself being drawn to reading books and listening to tapes that helped to empower and provide me with the answers I had been seeking. I continued having conversations in my mind and out loud with God. Finally, my fear stopped screaming at me, and when it quieted down, I realized the answers I had been searching for had always been there, but now I was able to hear them and to see them. I had a new perspective on life.

During my whole experience, I would have lightbulb moments, so to speak. I call them REALIZATIONS. These realizations take place in our life when our spirit starts to become aware of its SELF. It is a deep awareness, recognition, or insight into who we really are.

One of these insights happened when I was lying on my bed one day and an overwhelming feeling encircled me, and I felt how much I was loved. This sensation engulfed my entire body. This feeling let me know that I was truly loved by my family, my husband, and my friends. I never knew before this how much.

I became aware of how much I loved myself. Yes, you heard it right. I loved myself. I loved my power, my knowingness of Spirit, my ability to create, my humor, my sorrow, my circumstance, and my body. It took an experience like breast cancer to show me to myself.

I had many insightful moments come to me through this whole process. Another one of them was realizing I was not my body. Even if I had to have both breasts removed, I would still be me. I was much more than this physical shell and the material world around me. This realization helped me to stop comparing myself with other people as I had done in the past. It helped me to appreciate me, just the way I am. I had to release jealous thoughts, envy, and feelings of not being good enough.

Many times in the past, I would get upset and not speak for days to whomever I was with at the time. I would repeatedly have thoughts and dreams of people leaving me. One of my greatest fears throughout my life was being abandoned, being left because I wasn't good enough. I held these thoughts and emotions inside of me for years. I realized I had been carrying them around since I was a little girl. In fact, I realized I may even have held them in my consciousness before my birth.

Now, at the age of 37, I came to understand I was only hurting myself. I would come to know over time that these tiny little hurts in my heart, these thoughts and feelings I had would come to matter. *Literally*, they would become matter *(something solid or having form)*. This matter I am speaking about started to form a mass, and this mass formed inside of me. This is one reason when we are depressed, jealous, angry, or discouraged, people usually say, *"What's the matter with you?"* I had to start looking at WHY I was holding on to these negative emotions. I realized if I did not release them, they would keep building up inside of me.

Shortly after my experience, I was introduced to a book called *Abraham, A New Beginning II* by Jerry and Ester Hicks. This book is all about how our thoughts, words, and actions create our reality. It speaks about *well-being* and how it is our natural state of existence and flows to us at all times. It talks about the importance of *feeling good*. In fact, feeling good should be the most important aspect of our desires. I have read a lot of books in my lifetime, all geared around metaphysical studies, but this particular book resonated with me in a big way.

After reading this book, I realized going through breast cancer had already helped me to start to become aware of my thoughts! I was in the process of shifting my thoughts and beliefs about myself. I had been getting in touch with my emotions and how I wanted to feel. I did start to realize that all the "dis-ease" I carried around for years had manifested in my body as disease. Everything started to make sense.

I realized why forgiveness was important. When you forgive someone else or yourself, you release the resistance inside of you and allow your connection with *well-being* to flow. The energy of well-being is like water flowing through a hose. When you hold onto anger, unforgiveness, jealousy, hatred, envy, feeling not good enough, you are kinking up your own hose. You are putting a knot in your pipeline, and the stream of well-being can not flow freely through you. You are only hurting yourself.

After recognizing all of this, it became clear that I created my experience with breast cancer. I drew this situation to me. I realized I was not a victim of anything, but the creator of my experience. Every time I felt anger, rage, jealousy, or fear, I wasn't allowing my well-being. I was beginning to understand the power of my thoughts and beliefs. I needed to continue to stay conscious of the way they made me feel. I had to keep on recognizing my feelings each time before I could reach for better thoughts.

This was not something bad; in fact, this was awesome! God/Life was showing me what I needed to look at within myself. This was a gift!

In *Conversations with God, Book 1* by Neale Donald Walsch, it says, *"What you resist persists and what you look at disappears,"* meaning, when you push against or feel resistance toward something or someone, the situation or behavior will keep showing up in your life. If you really look at a situation or a person's behavior and become aware of what it is you are pushing against or feeling resistance toward, you can then change how you respond or react to it. The situation or the behavior will lose its power and disappear from your experience. This is how great God/Life is. Life is always giving us messages along the way and showing us to ourselves.

I began to understand if something or someone angers, frustrates, or discourages me, it only means I am holding onto something inside of me that needs to be looked at. I was not allowing my own well-being to flow! It was perfectly normal and okay for me to have negative emotions, but if I felt them on a consistent basis and did not release them, they would continue to build up inside of me.

The great news for me was, since I created my experience, I could recreate it. I could change my thoughts and beliefs about myself and allow my well-being to flow. I could focus on how wonderful my life is instead of focusing on how I wasn't good enough. I wanted to start loving myself again. I wanted to stay around as long as I could. I wasn't ready to go anywhere, anytime soon. I could be someone who had cancer who was fearful or I could be someone with cancer who was hopeful. I was changing my perspective about myself and about life.

I came to understand that my confusion, early on in my questioning whether I should or should not take chemo, was right on! The reason I had been confused about what to do is because it didn't matter if I had chemo treatments or not. Either way was okay. There was no right or wrong, only how I felt about taking the chemo and what I believed to be true for me.

After going through the whole experience, I made a decision that I wanted to comfort others along their path. Being faced with my own mortality somehow helped me to not fear death anymore. I had realizations that life goes on even after we leave this physical world. And this other place we go is called the nonphysical dimension. It is a place where we transition to when we depart this life. It is where our consciousness becomes one with the true essence of our creator. It is the most wonderful, loving place to go. It is not a bad thing; in fact, it is something to look forward to! I wanted to be of service to others and help them to feel assured and comforted in their last days on earth. So, I decided to volunteer my services and time to hospice patients, people who were ready to make their transitions. Funny how I thought I was comforting them, but they always ended up comforting me! I did that for a few years. It was very rewarding.

Each moment generates new circumstances for us all, but my life and the way I look at things have forever shifted. Cancer was the best thing that could have happened to me. I am now a Certified Life Empowerment Coach and my business, *Empowering Pathways, Universal Laws Life Coaching*, allows me to live my dream and my passion.

In my coaching practice, I help clients get whatever it is they want in their life. Life is supposed to be good. I also encourage, motivate, and support people going through any illness or disease and help them reclaim their natural state of health by becoming aware of their thoughts and feelings.

We do not have to go through life with illnesses and pain, but when illness is present, we can learn from it and turn suffering into wisdom. Life is supposed to be good. It is time for us all to live the life we deserve!

> ***"We are not creatures of circumstance,***
> ***we are CREATORS of circumstance"***
> —*Benjamin Disraeli*

Chapter 5
Mastering Your Thoughts and Feeling Good

Now, let's focus on you!

Take a look at your life, and you will find yourself there. Everywhere you go, there you are!

The first place to start is to fine-tune your desires in life. You need to become aware of what you are thinking on a daily basis.

I would like you to take a few moments to complete the following questions and write down your answers. Focus on the subject of **HEALTH** for the exercise.

1. What is it you **want** right now?

2. Why do you want it?

3. What current thoughts do you have about what you **want**?

4. How do these thoughts make you feel, and which thoughts feel better than others?

5. If they do not feel good, write down how you want to feel. If they feel good, skip to question 6.

6. Why do you want to feel this way?

7. What is something you could do to keep these thoughts active?

8. What does your desired goal or outcome look like?

Asking yourself these questions will help you to understand how you have been creating. Stop thinking about what you DON'T want and the reasons behind why you DON'T have it, and start thinking about what you **DO WANT** and **WHY** you want it. Then, start activating the new thoughts and feelings by talking about them and demonstrating them through your actions.

Some suggested ways to reinforce your thoughts,

feelings, words, and actions are through affirmations, visualizations, posting notes around your home or office, journaling, cutting out and making a collage of pictures about your desire, or meditating.

Here are some examples of negative thoughts versus positive ones and the difference between the two.

Negative *(not allowing the flow)*

- Everything goes downhill when you get older
- Everyone knows cancer can kill you
- My family has a history of cancer, so I was destined to get it
- I don't understand why this is happening to me
- I don't know what to do anymore
- Life is not fair

Positive *(allowing your well-being to flow)*

- I am like fine wine; I get better with age
- There are many people who have successfully triumphed over cancer
- I am my own person, and I create how I choose to feel

- I don't need to understand why I am experiencing this illness
- There are many things I still enjoy and love to do
- Life is good, and even though I feel bad now, it sure is nice to know well-being is my natural state

Take a moment and reflect how each of the negative and positive statements makes you feel. Create your own list of positive statements like the example given, and post these affirming thoughts everywhere you can!

When I mention the word *well-being* throughout this reading, I am talking about the essence of who you are. When you feel good, you are aligned with well-being. This is your true self.

All thought is vibration. When I mention the word vibration, it means the same thing as rhythm, pulse, or beat. Everything in the Universe has a rhythm; it pulsates, moves, and changes form. Law of attraction causes the same vibrations to come together, and then it produces an effect; this could be called *cause and effect.*

When you think a thought, you begin to feel, and when you feel, you send out energy that travels inside your body and outside of your body as well. This energy is a conscious energy. It attracts and produces an experience.

Everyone has a built-in guidance system, and it can help you navigate in the direction you *want* to go. It is exactly what it says it is—a *guidance system.* Start listening to it. It lets you know how you are feeling. This can be a challenge at times, because we have been taught throughout our life and in society to ignore our feelings. But, feelings are the language of your soul.

Negative emotion can be viewed as something positive. It means there is a strong desire for something you want, but the negative feeling is pulling you in the opposite direction of your desire. You will feel the emotion in your body. It is much more beneficial to try and refocus on something that helps you to feel positive emotion. You will then be moving in the direction of your desire and where you want to go, and you will be allowing the well-being to flow freely through you.

When I first learned this information, I started to become fearful of my thinking. Every time I had a negative thought, I was afraid it was going to manifest. I would like to take the pressure off you right now. This cannot happen. Most of us are not instant creators. It takes an extreme amount of focused energy directed at the same kind of thoughts and feelings to actually matter, to become matter. This is one reason cancer and other diseases often occur later in life. It takes consistent, resistant thoughts and beliefs being held in contrary to well-being, over a period of time, to manifest disease.

Negative emotion is a form of resistance; it is pushing against the stream of well-being. It is like rowing a canoe in the opposite direction of a rolling river. The water is flowing fast and you will eventually get to your desired place, but you will be exhausted and most likely sick. It is never too late to turn your canoe around and go in a much easier direction. Good feelings, thoughts, and beliefs will help you to feel better and align you with who you really are. They will place you in the calm of the river. You won't even need a paddle for your canoe; you can just go with the flow.

How do you get to these *good feelings* when you are depressed, afraid of a diagnosis, or feel bad about an illness?

- Become **AWARE** of your feelings
- **ALLOW** yourself to feel your feeling
- Feel the emotion fully

- Now have a conversation with yourself
- Start talking about what you are feeling, and then try to move the conversation in the direction of how you WANT to feel.

An example dialogue could be:

I am really down and I feel bad. I am scared to death about this illness I have. I hate that this is happening to me. It makes me angry that I have to go through something like this. God must really want to punish me. Life just doesn't go the way you want it to. I want this all to go away. There is only so much I can take, and it isn't easy going through this. Yeah, some days are better then others, but I am tired and ready to be done with this. It's hard to believe everything happens for a reason, but maybe that is true. I just haven't figured the reason out yet. Maybe I don't have to figure it all out. I believe somehow this whole experience is going to make me stronger. I want to feel better. I want to be myself again.

Did you notice how the dialogue shifted over time to a better feeling? What started out as depression and feeling bad ended up on a more positive note of wanting to at least feel better. This example is quite an extreme shift of vibration, and you may not be able to achieve this drastic of a change right away. That's okay. Even shifting from depression and fear to anger is a first step. Any relief you can give yourself is relief nonetheless.

Another example dialogue:

Today is not going to be a good day. I am already feeling overwhelmed and frustrated. I just don't have the energy. I have so much to do, and I don't know where to begin. I bet it will rain all day today. I should at least get dressed. I don't like feeling this way. I do have a lot on my plate at times, so it makes sense I would feel this way. I know I don't have to get it all done at once. After all, what is the worst that could happen? I could at least brush my hair and brush my teeth. Maybe I would feel better if I did that. I like the way my mouth feels after I brush my teeth. That usually perks me up. I know when I get dressed I usually feel a little better, too.

Did you notice the shift? This dialogue started with doubt/frustration and ended with optimism.

Every time you have a conversation with yourself, start becoming aware of how you are feeling with each thought you have. Then start talking to yourself out loud until you feel some relief. Make this a daily practice, even when you are feeling good. Start talking to yourself. People will think you have lost your mind. This would be a good thing. You have to lose your mind, so to speak, and connect with your heart!

Here is a metaphor you can use to remind yourself of how you are thinking:

Think of your thoughts as a freight train going down the track. See your desire of what it is that you are wanting as your destination or drop-off point. When you have negative thoughts that don't feel good, your train gets thrown off the track and its course. It wants to move ahead, but the wheels are not in alignment anymore. If you are detached from the track, you cannot get to your destination. *This is where having a conversation with yourself can be helpful.* Because in order to progress in the direction you want to go, picking up your train and repositioning it back on the track is the only way to move forward. Then, you can move full steam ahead. As you blast your horn with exhilaration, everyone around you will want to know how they can take part in your glorious ride. Some will stop and pull over and watch as you fly by them. They may even get aggravated and say you are getting in their way, but you will be sitting right up front in the conductor's seat, smiling and waving as you pass by. Once your train reaches its drop-off point, it continues on to the next one. This train never has a final destination. Its joy is always in the journey. It is the ultimate joy ride!

Become conscious of your dialogue. This is a VERY important first step. Have a conversation with YOU. You are your best friend. You are the only one who knows what you want. Eventually, you will be back on track with your desire and headed in the direction you want to go. You will be a conscious creator. You might even be called a *master* creator with a *master* mind!

I believe we are all masters. If we could begin realizing that our thoughts, feelings, words, and actions are creating all of our experiences, we would realize this really is and could be *A Wonderful Life!*

A great master creator was Walt Disney. He took thought beyond where it had ever been. He achieved his desire in life by visualizing and imagining with his mind. His attitude was positive, confident, joyful, and optimistic. I am sure he stayed mostly in the energy of hope and optimism and very little in doubt and fear. He aligned himself with well-being and allowed it to flow.

How do I know this? His manifestation is the proof.

There are many master creators walking on our earth today. There are many people whose wheels are aligned perfectly on the track of life and consciously manifest their desires most all the time and are living life to its fullest. They may not always know what lies around the next curve or bend, but they are aligned with well-being, and their train keeps moving full steam ahead.

Society sometimes tends to look at these people as greedy, dirty rich, damn lucky, stuck up know-it-alls who don't care about the little people. Many of these people are in this place of demonstration because they have allowed their well-being to flow. They are not attached to other people's opinions. Their thoughts and feelings will most likely be confident, fearless, expectant, optimistic, encouraging, and self-empowering. They have great desire and know exactly what they want out of life. At the same time, they are allowing and attracting it to come into their experience, and there is little resistance. What a glorious place to be.

"We have come forth into a world of contrast to give birth to our desires and to create them."
—Abraham Hicks, A New Beginning 11

My husband recently told me how Tiger Woods was trained to focus his attention when golfing on the golf course. His father would stand behind him with pots and pans and drop them on the ground as he was putting. He was trained and taught at a very young age how to focus his thoughts on what he wanted to achieve and how not to let outside circumstances affect his performance.

Norman Vincent Peale talks about a man he knew who was diagnosed with the worst cancer anyone could have and was told he only had a short time to live. The man could hardly believe it. One day he received a card in the mail from a friend, and it read, *"With God all things are possible."* After reading the card, the man was moved by the saying. The words empowered him, and he made a decision to start allowing his well-being. He began to visualize and use his imagination every day. He would visualize the cancerous cells being destroyed and new ones being replaced. He said *he did it with God and knew anything was possible.* The man did this repeatedly and, over a period of time, recreated his experience of cancer. His doctor was amazed at his results and later told him at an office visit that all the cancer was gone. This man lived a long, healthy, and happy life. This is the power of hope, optimism, and positive expectation. This is the power of your thoughts and beliefs!

When you begin mastering your thoughts and feeling good, you will be flying down the straightaway on life's never-ending tracks! It will be all you have ever dreamed of and much more!

> *"Our life is what our thoughts make it."*
> *—Marcus Aurelius*

Chapter 6
Loving Yourself,
Love in Your Self

I know you have heard the phrase *"You must love yourself first."* Well, I had heard it a million times and never understood what it was really supposed to mean. After my experience with breast cancer, the still, small voice within me was not whispering anymore—it was screaming. It spoke so clearly, it is one of the reasons I am writing this book.

Do you know what it actually means to love yourself? I am not speaking of loving your physical body, although that is important, too. I am speaking about a deeper connection beyond the physical shell you now reside in. Loving yourself means having a relationship with self and knowing that you are an important part of All That Is! You understand you are at one with God and not separate from God. It also means you are at one with love and not separate from love.

When you first meet someone, you want to know all about them and get to know them. You want to know their likes, dislikes, and values. You recognize when they are feeling good or when they are feeling bad. You come to respect, admire, and appreciate them. You support and encourage them. You go out of your way to accommodate them. How awesome would it be if you could do this for yourself?

When you start loving yourself, you will begin to understand that whatever you want to experience in life, such as love, joy, peace, abundance, or health, you must first embody it yourself. When you love yourself, you want to share your love with others. Love becomes an extension of who you are. You do not have conditions in a relationship because you know you are unconditional love.

If you do not love yourself, you could be attracting to you, at some level, the experience of cancer and possibly other illnesses, too. This is what my intuition and going through my experience has revealed to me. I do not claim to be an expert of any kind in the field of diseases. I am only sharing with you what I have come to understand from Spirit speaking to me through my own experience. It is one of the reasons so many women are affected with breast cancer. It is associated with our emotions and manifests itself in the chest area. You might say it is truly at the HEART of the matter!

When you hold in a lot of anger and feel unloved, not worthy, unattractive, extreme dislike for yourself, you are not in the flow with well-being. You are going in a different direction, and you are steering your train right off the track.

These insecure, uncomfortable thoughts and feelings we hold in our consciousness begin to send a signal and energy throughout the body. Over a period of time, Law of Attraction begins rounding up, gathering together, and summoning to you what you have been thinking and most importantly, what you have been feeling. You are sending out vibrations that are not in alignment with who you really are. If the "dis-ease" you've been feeling is not recognized, over time, it will begin forming a mass.

Amass (a mass) means to accumulate, collect, build up, hoard, assemble, store up, gather, and pile up. This is what you are doing to your body when you hold on to resistant thoughts and beliefs. They are accumulating, collecting, and building up inside of you. Once you are able to recognize and let go of these types of thoughts and beliefs by focusing on "what feels good" instead, then you will become a vibrational match with well-being.

Examples of this could be:

- I know I have a lot of great qualities vs. I hate the way I look
- I am just as worthy as anyone vs. I don't deserve good things
- I am a good person vs. I am no good
- I love myself vs. I hate myself
- I am a powerful creator vs. I am a victim of circumstances
- I can accomplish whatever I put my mind to vs. I am not smart
- I am attractive in many ways vs. I am ugly

Loving yourself can be of *grave* importance to your health. In fact, it should be the most important priority in your life.

There is great joy to be found, and it resides inside of you! When you are enjoying yourself, you have joy in yourself. When there is joy in your heart, you are full of joy; you are joyfully creating your experiences.

There are many great masters who walk the earth, and they are reading this book. Yes, it is you! You are a master, and you are a master creator. We are all master creators but have forgotten how powerful we are. Our core nature is love.

Destructive power comes from fear and not from love. When you fear something or someone, your reaction is to attack them or get defensive. This can take form through your thoughts, your words, or a physical attack on someone. When you are defensive in your outward actions, your body's reaction is to become defensive inwardly as well. Your words and actions, you might say, could be *aggressive*. Does this word sound familiar when thinking of cancer or disease? How many times have people been told their cancer is the "aggressive" type?

Become aware of the thoughts and beliefs you hold about yourself and about others. Ask yourself, "What do I love about myself?" If you feel negative emotion when you ask yourself that question, then begin focusing on the parts of yourself you do like. If you can't seem to find anything positive, then remind yourself of who you really are. You ARE love, spirit, eternal, pure positive energy, and you are powerful, whether you know it or not.

"With great power comes great responsibility" was a line in the movie *Spiderman*. My interpretation of what I believe this to mean is, when you are aware of who you really are as a spiritual being, there is great love, consistency, trustworthiness, reliability, and honesty in your character. It does not mean you are responsible for anyone else. It means you are in charge of yourself. You are only responsible for the love in yourself or *loving yourself*. When you love yourself, you become a mirror for the world, and others see themselves in you.

> *"Would you sell both your eyes for a million dollars…or your two legs…or your hands…or your hearing? Add up what you do have, and you'll find that you won't sell them for all the money in the world. The best things in life are yours, if you can appreciate yourself."*
> —*Dale Carnegie*

Here is an exercise that can help you to see your beauty, your true essence. It will help raise your energy level so that you can begin feeling good and letting in all that you deserve.

Ideally, you could tape this and then play it back.

I FEEL GOOD (Meditation)

Sit somewhere quiet. Close your eyes and relax. Breathe in slowly and deeply through your nose and out through your mouth. Visualize yourself and see yourself in your mind for a few moments.

Now, picture yourself standing in the middle of a large group of people. These people are all your friends or family. People you know or have known or people who have passed over. They love you very much. Feel their love pour down on you. Their love bathes you as if you were standing in a shower. Allow it to wash over you. Feel this love as much as you can. As it is cleansing you, you begin to feel refreshed and renewed.

You start to smile and notice how you are feeling and how you look when you smile. The people in the group admire you for all you are. There is no judgment about anything. You are the center of attention. You start to laugh and smile. Keep noticing how you are feeling. As you are laughing and smiling you start to send out a bright white energy field. Begin to see this energy. It is permeating each person in the group. You notice that they want to get closer to you. They begin smiling and laughing, too. You can feel their energy and it feels good. You realize the better you feel, the better they feel. And the better they feel, the better you feel. It is a wonderful energy exchange. You notice that there is nothing you have to do, have, or be. You are just yourself. You could live like this forever because it feels so good. In fact, you realize your true nature is to FEEL GOOD.

The whole group thanks you one by one, and you thank them for being there. You feel very energized and light. They ask you if you could come again whenever you need a boost of energy or a cleansing. They tell you how much they love to feel your happiness. You acknowledge them and say so long for now.

You can open your eyes and enjoy the feelings that you experienced from this exercise.

Chapter 7
Your Soul's Purpose

I f you have gotten this far in the book and are thinking, *Well, you know, this is all great and dandy, but how can I feel good about cancer, when someone I loved has died from it? Or, how about also, when I know I have it?*

First let me say, you have every right to feel the way you do, and it makes perfect sense for you to have this thought. It can be difficult to look at cancer in a positive light when you have it or may have had to witness and experience a long and grueling illness with someone you love. They may even have made their transition back into the nonphysical dimension.

If you are depressed, full of grief or despair from a

loved one's passing, allow yourself to fully embrace all of your feelings. There are several phases of grief that we go through, and each person may experience them differently.

Eventually, you will begin to activate the feeling of anger. Anger is a positive emotion when you have been feeling depressed or are grieving. Anger expressed can be a way of releasing the resistance within you, because if you feel powerless, anger can give you back some power, self- choice, and determination. With each feeling you go through, you will experience less resistance around your loved one's transitioning.

Your next emotion could be blame. Blame is less resistant than anger. Allow yourself to FEEL blame. Allow yourself to feel all your emotions. Embrace each one as you move through them. Eventually, it may take some time, but you will regain momentum and progress up the ladder of emotions to feeling joy, again!

In addition to all of this, I would like to say that death is an illusion; there is no death. We do not die. We are all *eternal,* powerful, spiritual beings. We are not these physical bodies we reside in. The bodies we're in are our coats, and when we are ready to take them off, we do. If you can embrace this thought about death, whether you have cancer or not, your entire life and the way you look at it can change in the twinkling of an eye. But don't take my word for it. Listen to your own feelings on this one and ask yourself how you feel when you hear this. Does it feel good or bad to know you are eternal?

Right now, you are physically focused here on this earth, but when you transition, you will come to know your own powerful, focused, eternal, creative, positive, conscious energy. This energy vibrates at the speed of light and exists at a very different frequency than that of the earth. It is pure positive energy. It is the highest form of love you can imagine or feel.

When you think of a loved one who has passed, you think of them as how you knew them when they were here on earth. You associate them with the behaviors, traits, disposition, and faults they may have had, but they are no longer those things. The unconstructive parts of the personality fall away, and the magnificent nature remains. When you think of them and you are sad, they are feeling wonderful, so it is not easy for them to join you in your sadness. They are pure positive energy. They are experiencing their true self. You must align your energy with theirs now. If you can embrace their transitioning and know they are perfectly happy, then you will be able to feel their presence again.

You can communicate with them at any time. You can even ask them to give you some type of sign that they are around. Then, stay open to whatever shows up. Electricity is one way your loved one may contact you. Examples of their presence could be seen as a lightbulb popping or going out, television screens turning on or off automatically, or through a song playing on the radio.

Look up the word electricity. You will find related words to be: power, current, energy, and force. Don't be surprised if the *force* is with you!

Before we come to this earth, we have a very clear desire and a full understanding and knowing of "the bigger picture." We all choose different environments, depending on the experience or desire we are reaching for. This is true for children and infants as well. It is through our thoughts and beliefs we recreate each time, how we experience the process. No two experiences are exactly the same.

Did you know we are all connected to each other? When you experience something, I have the ability to experience it, too. Someone who appears to suffer here on earth may be a catalyst in helping another shift their vibration to a higher level of thought and belief about themselves.

Let's take Christopher Reeve, for example. He was Superman. He could not overcome paralysis and made his transition back into nonphysical reality, but before he came forth on this physical plane, his soul had a desire it wanted to fulfill. He was always at choice on how to feel and how to move through his experience. He was a master creator. He took thought beyond where it has ever been. This means he made up his mind to make the best of his circumstance. He did not see himself as a victim. He embraced his circumstance and used his situation as a way of bringing awareness to others and raising funds for further research to the spinal cord injury community. I believe his soul had a much larger purpose, and his circumstance allowed him to be an instrument in accomplishing that. Many lives were changed because of his example. He helped people move to new thoughts within themselves about who they really are. I am sure his soul knew this on a very deep level of understanding. We should all be extremely grateful to have witnessed this incredible soul's life experience and his power of SELF or should I say SELFLESSNESS? Now, this is what I call a Super Man! His wife Dana was also a Super Woman!

Only the person having the experience knows! Your soul knows its purpose and why it is going through what it is going through. No one can say it should be this way or that way. Each soul has its own intention and knowing on a much deeper level than we understand. The point I am making is that staying here on the earth may not always be the outcome a particular soul chooses to experience.

When you have experienced the loss of someone you love to such a circumstance, take a moment and ask yourself:

- In what way has this person touched my life?
- What did I learn from their experience?
- What was I able to share or communicate to them that I might not have been able to otherwise?
- What were they able to share or communicate with me that they might not have been able to otherwise?
- What if you knew in your heart they were not gone forever and that you would see them again?
- What if you could look at this circumstance as being just what their soul chose to experience at a deeper level than you might understand right now?

And the most important belief to embrace is: **THEY DID NOT DIE**. They have returned to the full knowing of who they really are. They are pure positive energy; they are eternal and so are you.

Are you a caretaker for someone who is going through cancer and you are finding it difficult to deal with? Take a moment and ask yourself:

- What am I feeling?
- What am I afraid of?
- Why?
- How much of what I am feeling has to do with me?
- What is it I want to feel?
- Why?
- Have a conversation with yourself

An example dialogue could be:

I am feeling really sad about my sister's illness. I am afraid because I don't want her to leave me. How can I feel good when she is suffering so much? It doesn't seem fair. Things will be so different when she is gone. I don't want to be without her. I can't imagine my life any other way. I know she is in a lot of pain and my wanting to keep her here is more about me needing her and wanting her to stay. After all, we shared a lot together. It is okay to feel this way. I want to feel joy again when I am with her. I know our days are short together, and I realize when I am sad it most likely doesn't help her feel any better. I am doing the best I can for now. I know my sister has always had a great sense of humor. I want to feel happy again because I know that is what she would want for me. I would like that for me, too.

What you will find is that most of us feel guilt, sadness, anger, frustration, powerlessness, despair, and worry when someone we love is going through an illness. This is normal. It is very difficult to watch someone you love suffer, and it makes perfect sense that you would have these feelings. But what conversation could you have with yourself? How could you shift your vibration to a better feeling place? You are in charge of only your vibration! *You cannot create for the other person. You can only create for yourself!*

I know when I was going through my experience, I wanted people near me who were optimistic, hopeful, and positive. It was okay to be sad and angry once in a while, but when it feels as if you're drowning, it sure is nice to have someone by your side who knows how to resuscitate and breathe new life into you again! You might even say they are a *"breath of fresh air."*

"There is no end. There is no beginning. There is only the infinite passion of life."
—Federico Fellini

If someone you loved has passed on, here is an exercise to help you reconnect with them and to feel some relief around their transitioning:

COME INTO THE LIGHT (Meditation)

Sit in a comfortable place and close your eyes. Breathe in through your nose and out through your mouth a few times and relax.

Picture in your mind's eye your loved one standing in front of you. Take time to just visualize them for a few moments until you can see them clearly in your mind. Remember a happy time or a funny occasion you shared together. See them laughing and smiling in your vision. Feel the joy and love that is coming from them. See the love and joy as a stream of white light they are emitting, and it is penetrating into your being. Feel the energy. Allow the moment to be a silly, funny, joking, and happy time. Stay in this feeling place for as long as you want.

Ask them whatever you would like at this time. Let your intuition open up. Listen patiently for their answer. If you cannot intuit a response, then just BE with the person for awhile.

When you feel you would like to leave, give them a big hug and thank them for sharing their JOY with you. Let them know you would like to share this feeling again, whenever you feel it is necessary.

Do this exercise as often as you can. This is who they are now. This is their true essence. How you think about them and where they are will eventually start feeling better. This exercise will help you to raise your vibration, and you will be able to sense and feel them much more easily in your presence.

Chapter 8
New Desire and
a New Diagnosis

When you have been given a diagnosis from a doctor of any kind that seems bleak or discouraging, your guidance system will be speaking to you at this point loud and clear. It will be letting you know if what you have just heard feels good or not.

If it does not feel good for you to hear such news, then you should be listening to your guidance system and telling yourself this is a message to you that your doctor is not very hopeful or encouraging and is guiding you to a swift ending.

If your doctor has told you that you have something

that is terminal and you are dying, you should look him or her in the eye and say *"Aren't we all?"* No one's path is predestined. You can always make way for a new path in every moment. No one has the right to tell you where your path is taking you. After all, you are the creator of it!

Society has been holding the belief for a long time that when a doctor gives you a negative diagnosis, it is an unchangeable reality. You begin to believe it can be no other way. Do you believe they know more than your own body and spirit? How does it feel to hand over your power to someone else? Do you really think they know more about your destiny than you?

When you hear bleak news of any kind from a doctor and they tell you your path has been chosen, tell them that is never really true of anyone. Thank them for their grim consultation and let them know what is really happening—the contrast is giving you a new, strong desire. Tell them an awareness is being born within you, and because of this news, you will have a powerful summoning of life moving through you and that they should be so lucky! Tell them "thank you," and leave the office. If your doctor says, *"I am just telling you like it is,"* then tell him or her you are going to focus on a new desire and a new diagnosis. Tell them you are

going to focus on *"what could be"* instead of *"what is!"*
Doctors should be a bridge of hope, encouragement, and optimism. They should be holding the light when you are walking down what seems to be a dark and lonely road ahead. If they cannot hold the light, then you grab it and hold it for yourself!

Most doctors or medical people will have a hard time reading and understanding this type of thought. They are dependent on you and your sickness to keep them in business. It is what their whole life has been focused around. It is what their whole thought system has been conditioned to believe. It is, in fact, the majority of our society's beliefs that we need doctors to cure us.

I believe it is a **combination** of a positive, optimistic, encouraging doctor *and* our beliefs about who we are and the power within ourselves to heal, no matter what the diagnosis is.

I am sure most doctors and medical people care deeply for their patients and have only the best intentions for them. However, some doctors believe they know more than the person who is going through the experience because they have been to "Medical School" and have a degree. They believe they know more because of what they have seen and experienced in their training. They look at the *facts* and *statistics* and believe mostly in their observations. They will tell you that statistics have shown something to be true, but what they don't realize is that statistics are also the results of others dominant thoughts and beliefs! They look at "what is," instead of looking at "**what could be.**" They tend to make patients feel powerless over their situation instead of encouraging them to foster positive thoughts and feelings.

Most doctors would say they don't want to give their patients false hope, but what they don't realize is **HOPE** *is* the bridge that is crucial. In fact, there is no such thing as *false hope*; the two words contradict each other.

How can you cross an aggressive and raging river with ease unless there is a bridge that helps take you to the other side? We can be that bridge for people. We can hold the light of hope for them when they can not hold it for themselves. We can do for others what we would want done for us if we were in the same position.

Did you know Jesus did not see people as being sick! He knew well-being flowed to them at all times and all they had to do was let it in. They healed themselves by believing in him. When people were near Jesus, they FELT a presence. The presence they felt in Jesus was *FAITH, HOPE, and LOVE;* therefore, *FAITH, HOPE, and LOVE* were felt within them, through him. He held the light for them. He was a light unto the darkness and he cursed it not! He did not curse disease because he did not see it as a curse. He believed a healing could occur in a person's life, if they chose for it to be that way and that they may have been suppressing a significant number of negative thoughts and feelings within their mind and body. These thoughts and feelings had manifested in their body, and by believing they could be healed, they would free up the resistance and actually heal themselves! The message Jesus was trying to convey was, if you cannot let go of the resistant thoughts and beliefs yourself, then believing in him and the things that he did would be sufficient. Jesus helped us to get back on track! Patients who "believe" in their doctor's ability and in their advice usually regain their health.

Jesus was a master creator, and he held the light for many people. *He brought only tidings of comfort and JOY!* Jesus vibrated at a very high level of consciousness. He was pure positive energy in human form. These things that he did, we also can do! Sound familiar?

Pay more attention to the way you feel and start reaching for thoughts that feel good, thoughts that give you *FAITH, HOPE, and JOY.* Make a new decision to pamper yourself, adore yourself, and soothe yourself in every way you can.

Doctors are a great gift to us here on earth, and we **must** make use of their services, expertise, and knowledge, but do not frighten yourself by going for constant diagnosis. Soothe yourself into well-being by doing all your favorite things in life. Turn your attention away from what makes you feel bad and focus on what feels good! Create a new desire for yourself to live life to its fullest, the way it is really supposed to be, the real message Jesus was saying all along.

"As long as we have hope, we have direction, the energy to move, and the map to move by. We have a hundred alternatives, a thousand paths and infinity of dreams. Hopeful, we are halfway to where we want to go; hopeless, we are lost forever."
—*Hong Kong Proverb*

The following three chapters give a metaphorical glimpse into various perspectives that could connect with your particular situation or whatever you are going through. My intention is that you will find meaning and value within each of them—that you will identify with them and extract what feels good for you!

Chapter 9
The Key

An interesting incident happened to me when my husband and I moved my 18-year-old son into his first apartment for college. There is an amazing message that was revealed to me, in blocks of thought, days after it happened.

The day had arrived when my son, Shaun, was ready to move into his first apartment for college. It was a beautiful, picturesque Monday morning in sunny Florida when three broad-shouldered and powerfully built movers arrived at our front door ready to haul off furniture. Their attitudes were impressive, considering everything we had to move was up and down a lengthy flight of stairs.

My son eagerly hopped into his car without hesitation about leaving home, and his dad and I followed behind.

When we reached our final destination, we parked the car and checked into the front office of the apartment complex. I had been preparing for this move for over six months, and the manager of the apartment complex knew me quite well. She informed us that Shaun needed to fill out leasing papers and that my husband would have to stay with him and sign them, too, since he was the guarantor of the lease. She said it would take about 15 minutes to fill out and go over all the rules.

I knew we were paying the movers generously by the hour so I asked the manager to give me the key so I could let them start unloading the furniture. She asked me to *please not lose it* because they didn't have many keys to give out. I stated to her assuredly that the key would be in safe hands, thanked her, and then proceeded to my car.

I signaled the movers to follow me around to the apartment. I was anxious and excited to see the place. I had not seen this particular apartment until that day.

The apartment was located on the second floor. I parked my car and scurried eagerly up the stairs. My car keys, cell phone, and the apartment key were all in hand.

The door was wide open to the apartment, so I proceeded inside. I was greeted by a couple of sweaty maintenance men whose expressions glared at me with a frazzled pressure to meet a deadline. One of them was hanging on a ladder, installing and repairing a ceiling fan. The other maintenance man had all the horizontal blinds from the windows tossed out across the floor. All the kitchen door cabinets were disconnected from their brackets, the apartment was sizzling hot because the air-conditioning was not working properly, the washer and dryer were not where they were supposed to be, and the toilet in one of the bathrooms wasn't even attached to the ground. It became visibly apparent that the apartment was still in disarray and not ready for a tenant.

One of the sweaty maintenance men glared up at me and said, "Ma'am, this apartment is not ready yet."

"WHAT DO YOU MEAN NOT READY?" I snarled.

This was not acceptable. I was furious.

One of the things I was specifically angry about was that the girl who showed us the model apartment six months ago said the washer and dryer would be on the inside, down the hall. As it turned out, the washer and dryer were located outside in a porch closet, which was supposed to be used for storage.

I could feel my emotional state dropping. I went from enthusiasm and optimism to anger and rage in about three seconds. I was getting mad, and everyone around me knew it.

Meanwhile, the movers already had the couch in hand and were standing behind me asking where I wanted them to place it.

I told the maintenance men they needed to finish up and fast! I was beside myself at this point, so I phoned my husband for some assistance.

My hands were holding the car keys, cell phone, and apartment key. So, before I could dial my phone, I needed to free up my hands. I reached down and slid the apartment key into my right pocket and proceeded to call my husband. I asked him to get over here as soon as possible. I was not happy, and the apartment was NOT what I was expecting.

He knows when I am mad, and this was one of those times! He told me they were still busy in the office. I slammed my cell phone closed, still furious.

I remembered the manager instructing me not to lose the key to the apartment. So I reached in my right pocket just to check if it was still there.

It was GONE! I lost the key! I could not find it anywhere. I searched both pockets, but nothing. Panic set in, and the movers noticed I was feeling even more irritable and frustrated. They asked me if maybe I had dropped the key outside when I went to my car. They offered to help me look for it.

I checked my purse, and then we walked the grounds and the entire apartment for at least half an hour searching for the missing key. We rummaged around the grounds only to seek out garbage and other paraphernalia left behind by other tenants.

I continued to stay angry and kept focusing on the washer and dryer being on the outside porch instead of down the hall. I was considering not taking the apartment, but the movers had already moved in all the furniture. One of them helped me to shift my energy to a better feeling place by saying, *"You know teenagers could care less where their washer and dryer are located anyway."*

He was right; most teenagers really wouldn't care.

After he said that, I began to realize how my anger and frustration were kinking up my hose. I was not letting in my desire for finding the key. So, I began to do some self talk. I started a dialogue with myself, a conversation that would shift my thinking.

I started to say things like, *"You know, at least Shaun has a place to stay. It could be a lot worse. I am happy my son wants to go to school. I know getting angry isn't helping this situation. He must be excited about living on his own and being independent. He probably doesn't even care where the washer and dryer are located. It doesn't feel good to be angry. I want to feel good. I want Shaun to see me happy. I want this to be a good experience for him. He is going to love this place. I know if I relax I will find the key somehow."*

Believe it or not, I started to feel a lot better after some self talk.

I started to relax and enjoy setting up the furniture and fixing the apartment. I was beginning to have fun and looked forward to Shaun seeing his new place.

But, I still needed to find the key.

I reached into my pocket for one last check, and there it was.

THE KEY! I had FOUND the KEY. It was in my pocket. The key was right there in my pocket. I could hardly believe it.

The movers knew something great had happened. We were all thrilled and started jumping up and down with joy. They were just as happy as I was in finding the key.

My husband and son finished signing all the leasing papers, and when they arrived they both loved the apartment.

It turned out Shaun didn't care where the washer and dryer were. In fact, he liked it even better outside on the porch. He loved the place and was excited to get settled in. The rest of the day went extremely well. When we were ready to leave, we gave our son a big kiss good-bye and we headed back home.

The next few days passed, and I was visiting with a friend. She was complaining about her day and how horrible it had been. She was telling me how everything had been going wrong and how angry and frustrated she was getting. As she was talking, I thought to myself, too bad she just doesn't find some better feeling thoughts about this day. She needs to shift her vibration.

All of a sudden, I had a realization! I realized what had happened with the key episode. The message that came to me was "THE KEY" had been there ALL ALONG! We always have the key on us. When we get angry, frustrated, worried, etc. we LOSE ourselves and we lose the key. When we lose sight of our emotions, it becomes extremely difficult to find our key. The key is always there; we just have to relax, reach for better feeling thoughts, and try to feel good—then we will have better access to the *key*.

The key stood as a symbol and a sign of the power we all have inside us. We can unlock, unleash, and release our negative emotion at any time. We have the ability and the power to consciously, deliberately, and intentionally recognize when we are in a negative emotion. We can reach for better dialogue with our thoughts, turn the key, and open up a new point of view.

What an enormous lesson this was for me. I felt compelled to share it with you; it shows how powerful we really are. And this is the KEY message!

Chapter 10
Your Personal
Computer

Do you have a personal computer at home? Most of us do. Did you know you are very much like your computer?

People talk about the world being taken over by computers one day. What I believe this to mean is WE ARE the computers! Our world could be taken *over* by us! We have huge INPUT on how our life experience plays itself out. We can *enter* in exactly what we want. In fact, we are always inputting what we experience in our lives right now, all of the time. We're just not doing it on a *conscious* level.

Here is an example.

Just like your computer at home, the hard drive represents your mind. The keyboard represents your thoughts and beliefs. The monitor/screen displays what you enter in (your body), and the printer gives you an experience. The printer prints out your created work. They all perform together to give you your end result.

When you sit down at your computer to work or play, do you type in what you DO NOT want or what you DO WANT? Most likely, you type in what you want to find out, discover, or create.

This is the same process you do with yourself. Your hard drive (mind) supplies the energy for your computer (your self). When you think a thought or observe something, you enter it in on your keyboard (body).

It then shows up on your monitor/screen and replicates itself out as an experience in your life.

When there are too many programs running at the same time, your computer has a tendency to crash. And when you download programs that are damaging or open up harmful files, your computer is at risk for viruses! Does any of this sound familiar? How comparable are your body's reactions to these same descriptions?

What programs do you have running on your

computer? What programs would you like to delete or do away with? Are you installing what you want or what you don't want? What is showing up on your monitor screen, and what kinds of results are being printed out? Do you find you get a lot of viruses? Are you happy with what you are programming into your personal computer? If not, then maybe it is time to reboot and restore and begin putting in or downloading what you want!

Just like computer chips, your *cells* have memory and they store what you entered on your keyboard. When you shut down your computer and then turn it back on, it still retains memory. In the same way, your cells retain memory, too.

If you ingest something into your body that is foreign, your cells recognize it as something different and acclimate themselves to receive it. Your cells get used to whatever it is you are introducing to them. Down the road, when you think about the particular thing you had consumed and consume it again, it triggers the memory in the cells. They remember the food or drug you had ingested before. They adjust themselves accordingly. If they are given the same thing several times, they will begin asking for it. This is how cravings can occur. Our cells are amazing. They compensate for us all the time in whatever way we need them to.

All it takes to reprogram your personal computer is to change your thoughts and introduce what you want into your body instead of what you do not want. Over time, cells will assimilate and activate the thought and encode themselves with the new belief. This sounds easier said than done, but it can be done and has been done!

Let's take the example of the chemotherapy I had injected in my body for breast cancer. If I had approached this situation with the thought of the chemo being poison and toxic as it flowed through my body, then I would be entering that thought in on my keyboard (body). My cells would receive the input, then download and begin to activate the thought. If I were to hold that thought over a period of time, it would become a dominant thought and the cells would store memory of it. It would be an installed program. The program would show up on my screen, and then my printer would have printed it out as my experience. I would have experienced exactly what I believed and felt to be true. I would be playing the game I had installed. My cells would have done their best to play the game with me. I would have experienced the chemo as a poison and toxin going through my body. They would have done their job and reacted to the poison.

Our thoughts can be our healing or our suffering, our freedom or our bondage. Become aware of what games you are playing and what you are programming in on your computer! The good news here is, in most cases, you can uninstall the game at any time and download a new one.

"Change your thoughts and you change your world."
—*Norman Vincent Peale*

Chapter 11
The Wizard of
Ahhh Ha's

The power to create whatever you want in your life lies within YOU! This statement played itself out in the movie *The Wizard of Oz*. I love this movie and believe that this musical has some very spiritual messages in it.

It invites you to take a deep look into your imagining and dreaming mind and how powerful it can be. The mind can make known, bring to light, and manifest whatever it can dream or imagine. The mind is a powerhouse full of possibilities.

The movie showed that certain people are placed on

your path in life to help you along and help you to become the person you are today. Each person plays a particular role. Some people are with you for the entire journey, and some are only with you for a short time.

The Wicked Witch represented facing your fear. There will always be unpleasant people and circumstances that you come up against along your path, but you must keep moving forward. The people and circumstances have no power over you unless you allow them to! What you label as bad, evil, or wicked was actually placed there by you to help you step into your real power of self.

Glinda the Good Witch represented your higher self. She stood as part of your essence that knows only goodness and love. She portrayed the light within you that shows up in times of darkness.

People were convinced the tornado actually carried Dorothy and Toto away to an enchanted reality. It was a place, a real truly live place that existed somewhere over the rainbow. At least that's what people thought until they found out Dorothy had been dreaming all along. For Dorothy, the whole experience was real. In fact, she found it impossible to accept that she had been dreaming the whole time.

For those who are reading this who have cancer and

are now facing so-called "reality," I challenge you to take a closer look at what you label as reality. I quote the word "reality" because your reality is always changing. Just like Dorothy, if you want to experience a new reality, then you have to dream it into being. You have to imagine it as real. For your reality to become *real* depends only on how you choose to perceive it. Think about what I just said. If you view something as *real,* then it will be your experience of it, for sure!

The Scarecrow thought he was a failure because he didn't have a brain. Most people can relate to this character. People often think they are not good enough or smart enough. They don't give themselves the credit they deserve. The Scarecrow found out through his experience that he was able to reason and create the whole time. All the other characters believed in him— he just didn't believe in himself.

The Tin Man struck a chord with people because he thought he was imperfect. He wanted a heart to experience real emotions such as love, kindness, and sentimentality. He was out of touch with his feelings. Water represents emotion, so whenever he cried or it rained, the character would get rusty. He needed the oil from the oil can to release his resistance. The encounter he had with the other characters along the Yellow Brick

Road helped him express his feelings and register his emotions.

The Cowardly Lion thought of himself as a great big coward. He was afraid of stepping out of his comfort zone. He had to face his fear. When he finally stood up for himself and what he wanted, his fear started to lose power over him. It lost its grip, so to speak, and he discovered confidence and courage. He realized there was nothing to fear but fear itself. He became the King he was always meant to be!

Dorothy was in a state of forgetfulness. Everyone seemed familiar to her and she couldn't remember why. She needed to be awakened! Her journey to Emerald City helped her to face life's challenges and remember how much she was loved by the people that had always surrounded her.

The Wizard symbolized control and power. He believed he had power over everyone. He wasn't coming from a place of integrity. He hid behind a curtain and manipulated and intimidated those who approached him. He was the great and powerful OZ. All the characters believed in a power greater than they were. They were disillusioned in the end to discover that the Wizard of Oz wasn't a wizard at all. He was just like they were. This was the great AHHH HA! Once it was revealed that he was like everyone else, it discredited him and brought him back to reality. The Wizard of Oz was a good man at heart and realized he could help others by just being himself. Once he unveiled himself and stepped out from behind the curtain, he was free. He was so free he drifted away in the air balloon, leaving Dorothy behind.

Have you used power and control to intimidate others? Have you ever felt others were better than you? Have you been hiding behind your own personal curtain? How many times have you had to prove yourself worthy to someone? How would it feel to free yourself from those types of thoughts? How would it feel to know you're worthy regardless of what anyone may think of you?

Dorothy's ruby slippers were placed in front of her feet, and she stepped into them. This was symbolic for "stepping into your power." They also represented the ability to be able to connect back with what is important to you at any time.

Dorothy missed the air balloon ride back to Kansas, only to discover that the power to return home had been with her all along. She learned to appreciate life on earth and the people and loved ones who were with her.

The characters conquered the Wicked Witch, who

represented our fears in life. After completing their mission to defeat the wicked witch, they were able to comprehend their power. This would not have been understood completely if it weren't for the confrontation. They had to *experience* who they were!

What is it you have to confront and conquer to know who you really are? How can your experience empower you? What similarities from these characters do you see in yourself? Are you more like Dorothy, The Scarecrow, The Tin Man, The Cowardly Lion, or the Wizard?

Most all movies have a deeper meaning in them. Ask yourself next time you watch a movie, what message is it trying to get across? What deeper meaning could I extract from it? What is it mirroring to me? What could I learn from this?

If you ever have to go looking for your heart's desire, remember it is in your own backyard!

There is a magic potion that resides inside of you. Just like Glinda the Good Witch told Dorothy at the ending of *The Wizard of Oz*, "You don't need to be helped, you have always had the power!"

Chapter 12
I Am Positive

Remember, you are not a victim of circumstances but a creator of your circumstances. All experiences you go through are opportunities for you to look at how you are creating. They are showing you to yourself.

People along your path are angels in disguise and start becoming aware of who is playing a role in your life.

Feeling good should be the most important factor in the creating of your desires. It is not just about being positive; it is about actually having the feelings inside to match your attitude.

Keep your wheels on the track so your train can

travel effortlessly on its journey. If you steer yourself off your track, just realign and continue on.

Loving yourself is important. In fact, it is of grave importance. It could mean your life. When faced with breast cancer, it is at the heart of the matter!

Each soul has a purpose. And before you come forth onto this physical plane you have a greater knowing, a purpose and intent to create whatever it is that you desire. And no one can create in your experience but you!

Focus on what you want instead of what you don't want. Hope is crucial under any circumstance. You are the creator of your experience.

I shared with you a personal story of how you always hold the *key*. The key to how you want to feel. And it is this key that will unlock and let in everything you want to find. This key is available at any time.

I drew a comparison between you and your computer and how you should become aware of what you are entering in on your keyboard and what programs you have running.

I reminded you of how "you have always had the power." It is within you at all times. This is the great AH HA!

Having received all this information, what next?

How do you incorporate it all into your present experience?

It may seem hard to understand, and you may even feel overloaded by it all. If that is the case, just know it is normal. You have permission to shut down your computer and process it all.

If you have forgotten everything you have read so far, and it is just too much information to retain, then please remember this one point I am about to make.

The most valuable and significant message for you to take from this book is to start *lightening up*. Start having more fun! We all take life way too seriously. Life is supposed to be fun. You did not come here to suffer or experience disease. You came here to experience freedom, love, and joy.

Having fun is different for everyone. What is fun for one person may not be fun for the next. Do what feels good for you.

What exactly does fun look like? Here are some examples:

- Go for a bicycle ride
- Take a vacation
- Watch a comedy
- Take a walk

- Treat yourself to a massage
- Go out to lunch with a friend
- Play a favorite sport
- Put on dance music and dance in front of a mirror
- Go out dancing
- Buy a joke book
- Make silly faces in the mirror
- Run with your dog/play catch
- Wrestle on the floor with your children
- Play board games/cards
- Do impersonations of people you know
- Take a creative class
- Draw silly pictures
- Hike in the mountains
- Go swimming
- Go to the beach
- Get a manicure/pedicure
- Get your hair done
- Go to the zoo
- Write a book
- Write poetry
- Sing karaoke

Do what you love to do. See the humor in life.

Laughter is the best medicine. It literally allows your well-being to flow.

I am learning that we will never know it all anyway, and who really cares if we do? It doesn't matter who knows more, has more, or who has done more. We are in the process of becoming more in every moment.

Your life is what you make it to be.

When you are faced with a disease of any kind, remember God, love, joy, abundance, health, and all the things that equal well-being are with you at all times; your only job is to let it in! That is where the saying *"Let go and let God"* comes from. It means release negativity, worry, and ego, and let God in. Ease up on yourself, especially when you don't feel good. It is perfectly fine to feel all your emotions. Make peace with where you are. Go with the flow!

In closing, let me say **CONGRATULATIONS**, you are on the way to reclaiming your natural state of health. For you to be attracting this information says you have a desire to want to know more, and Law of Attraction is answering your request. You are a powerful creator!

There is a saying: *"I would have done better if I would have known better."* Now knowing what you know, you can start giving birth to new desires and your new self. You may even call it being born again!

Reach for the highest thoughts, the grandest feelings, and the best possible actions!

Let the sun shine in!

You can do it! I know you can, in fact, **I AM POSITIVE!**

Inspirational Poetry
by Leslie Bishop

The Calm

The mind is like water in a lake or a pond; at times it encounters storms and gets ruffled, but returns to the calm and peace of what it really is. And where murkiness lay present, now exists transparency.

The Dance

Peace plays beautiful music as turmoil tries to tempt her with his tune.

Her peace cannot be moved, her partner is strong.

As they dance and twirl in a frenzied embrace, it is within the rhythm they become one.

The Wall

You have built a wall through which your brother cannot enter

You look over your wall and see but one perspective

Why do you limit your sight, when beyond the wall is paradise?

The Spider

I am entangled in a web from which there is no escape.

I stay silent until my prey enters in.

My attack on this predator is my own cry for help.

Is there no escape?

Help me free myself from this thinned moss.

It cannot imprison me as I think it can.

I am the creator of this house.

Surely, I must know how to escape my own creation!

Gratitude

As I gaze out into the world I am filled with gratitude.

I am grateful for all things bestowed upon me.

What more could I ask for, but only that I may love more!

Who Am I?

I looked into the light and what did I see?

An image of myself for the light reflected me.

The love was great the love was grand and oh, how much I knew,

In the light was love and completeness too!

I bathed myself within the light and felt forever peace,

And in the moment knew freedom and release.

I promised I would stay and never wander far, but the light spoke to

My heart and said, "You cannot run from what you are!"

Bio:

Leslie Bishop is a Certified Empowerment Life Coach through the Institute for Professional Empowerment Coaching, who has spent the majority of her life training, teaching, and gaining knowledge in the field of metaphysical studies. Overcoming breast cancer herself, Leslie is a speaker and facilitator who coaches people going through illness or disease, and helps them create wellness by becoming aware of their thoughts and feelings. Leslie has introduced the Laws of Attraction to many people.

Contact Information for the Author:

If you would like additional guidance and support from the material you have read, or to become a coaching client, please feel free to e-mail: Lbsands@aol.com

Notes:

My sources for the quotes in this book have been many and varied. Two main books I have mentioned throughout the dialogue have been:

A New Beginning II, by Jerry & Ester Hicks. For more information go to www.Abraham-Hicks.com

Conversations with God, Book I, by Neale Donald Walsch. For more information go to www.cwg.org

Recommended Readings:

Louise L. Hay. *You Can Heal Your Life,* www.hayhouse.com

Bruce D. Schneider, Ph.D. *Relax You're Already Perfect*

Eckhart Tolle. *The Power of Now*

Ester & Jerry Hicks. *Ask and it is Given (The teachings of Abraham)*

Betty J. Eadie. *Embraced by the Light*

Jane Roberts. *Seth Speaks*

Neale Donald Walsch. *Home with God (In a Life That Never Ends),*

Conversations with God Books II & III, Friendship with God (an uncommon dialogue), Communion with God

Paul Ferrini. *I am the Door*

Exercise:

Bikram Yoga: www.bikramyoga.com

Information for the American Cancer Society:

1-800-ACS-2345 (1-866-228-4327) or
www.cancer.org